RICHES IN EDEN

Unlocking the Healing Power of God's Provision
in Nature

Emma M. Emmanuel

Riches in Eden

Unlocking the Healing Power of God's Provision in Nature

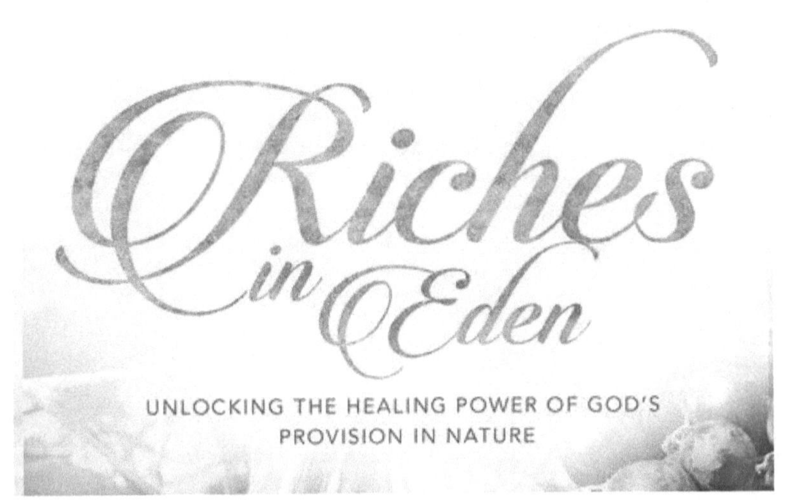

Emma M. Emmanuel

Dedication

To Jehovah God my Papa, my everything. You make all things possible.

To my wonderful children Renua, Aig, Ehi & Zara, for being my constant source of joy! I love you all more than you know.

To my parents, Emmanuel & Philomena Ofong-Ekpe, for loving me unconditionally.

To my sister, Stella Okuzu for always being there.

God bless you all!

Table of Contents

THE WORD

Is there no balm in Gilead; is there no physician there? Why then is not the health of the daughter of my people recovered?

Jeremiah 8:22

Down the middle of the great street of the city. On each side of the river stood the tree of life, bearing twelve crops of fruit, yielding its fruit every month. And the leaves of the tree are for the healing of the nations.

Revelation 22:2

I believe I have been commissioned to use my simple knowledge of home remedies to bring healing to the lives of people.

The words 'Is there no Balm in Gilead; is there no physician there; why then is not the health of the daughter of my people recovered?' was the first wakeup call I received after a workshop I delivered for a group of women on Gods provision for us in Nature.

For a long time, I felt like a 'Jonah' running away from my calling but now, I am ready to share my collection of write-ups and articles on what God has given us to self-heal.

Each weekend try out a new recipe! This book is not all recipes; there is also helpful information on lifestyle changes you can take on board.

This little book will reveal to you the Balm of Gilead sitting in your kitchen cupboard! Enjoy!

INTRODUCTION

In Genesis 1:29 God said, "I give you every seed-bearing plant on the face of the whole earth and every tree that has fruit with seed in it. They will be yours for food".

The online Dictionary defines food as:

'Any nutritious substance that people or animals eat or drink, or that plants absorb, in order to maintain life and growth.'

You can be sure that if God gives you food, that food is good. If we eat the food given to us by our heavenly Father, we will not even need to treat any ailment because we will be walking in good health

What we need to note is that food does not go into our bodies through the mouth only. Our bodies can be fed through the pores of our skin.

Ideally, our skincare products should be free from synthetic chemicals and harmful ingredients.

It is important that we take the time to read the ingredients of any product that goes on our skin as it eventually ends up in our blood stream. The way you read the nutritional contents of your food items when you go grocery shopping is what is expected when shopping for skincare products. Educate yourself on the ingredients contained in these products.

EVERYTHING GOD CREATED HAS A PURPOSE

Every plant has a purpose.

I believe and I have consistently said that God would not leave us on this planet (with all the problems He knew we would encounter) without providing the solutions to every problem we would come across.

Our God is an all-knowing God; and because our God is all-knowing, He knew Adam would fall. With Adams fall came curses.

The fruit from the trees in the garden were filled with Gods goodness. The tree in the middle of the garden brought death. That is the simple reason why we suffer ill health and physical death today.

Our all-knowing God knew the repercussions that would follow the fall.

However, even with the knowledge that man would fall, God still loved us so much that He had proactively provided all that we would need to take care of ourselves as we journey towards restoring our relationship with Him here on earth. He did not create the medicinal properties in the plants after the fall of Adam; they were already there even before Adam needed them.

First, we need knowledge. We need to know what is out there. The Bible says in Hosea 4:6 'My people are destroyed for lack of knowledge' Meaning that with knowledge, we are free from destruction.

I hope this book helps you acquire some life-giving knowledge.

Emma M. Emmanuel

NOURISHING FOODS

Natural foods are packed full of vitamins, minerals and anti-oxidants that our bodies need to stay healthy. The skin is the body's largest organ. As our bodies absorb into our bloodstream 60% of what our skin comes in contact with, the best thing you can do for your skin is to feed it these vitamins, minerals and anti-oxidants too.

Any food that is good for your health will generally be good for your skin too. Oils such as Avocado, Grapeseed Oil, Olive Oil, Sweet Almond Oil, Coconut Oil, Shea Butter Oil, Carrot oil and Rosehip are all nutrient rich oils packed full with vitamins and minerals for your skin and general well-being.

Other such nutritious herbs and foods are:

- Aloe Vera helps treats sunburn, is a moisturizer, treats acne, fights aging, treats gum disease etc.
- Myrrh has cancer-fighting properties, is antifungal, slows down the ageing process of the skin etc.
- Green Tea with antioxidants for skin repair
- Ganoderma (the reishi mushroom) FOR LONGEVITY
- Avocado with skin rejuvenating Vitamin E
- Carrots with Vitamin A for healthy vibrant skin
- Tomatoes for Lycopene which helps protect skin from UV rays
- Onions (red onions particularly) are packed full of Quercetin, which helps fight cancer and helps with hair growth
- Lemon rich in Vitamin C which is a natural deodorant, it helps combat body odour and is a natural skin lightener. Lemon also helps to cleanse the digestive system if taken first thing in the morning in warm water
- Flaxseed oil for the omega 3 fatty acids for skin repair

- Honey has great healing, antiseptic, cleansing and skin rejuvenating properties
- Olive oil is as a great cleansing agent and it nourishes and moisturises the skin.
- Palm oil is rich in vitamin E and Vitamin A. It has 15 times more Carotenoids than carrot oil and it help fight signs of aging on the skin.
- Yoghurt rich in Vitamin D is good for acne
- Garlic, apart from being good for your heart, helps with hair loss. God knew that with all the stress we would face our hair would fall off! Therefore, He put in place a solution for that!

The list goes on and on with all that He has put out there for us.

These foods and herbs were used in the Bible for the purposes God put them there for.

John 19: 39 - And there came also Nicodemus, which at the first came to Jesus by night, and brought a mixture of myrrh and aloes, about a hundred-pound weight.

Esther 2:12 - Before a young woman's turn came to go in to King Xerxes, she had to complete twelve months of beauty treatments prescribed for the women, six months with oil of myrrh and six with perfumes and cosmetics.

2 Kings 20:7 - Then Isaiah said, "Prepare a poultice of figs." They did so and applied it to the boil, and he recovered.

A GOOD SHINE AND POLISH

I remember as a child, on Saturday mornings, my father would give his car a good wash. After the wash, he'd spend the rest of the day waxing and polishing it. He had different little tin jars with different coloured felt cloths for each jar. The TLC paid off because after a while, you could only tell the age of the car from its number plate!

Thankfully we don't have number plates but if we don't start now to give our skin some TLC, our skin could easily become our number plates!

This weekend, we are going to give our skin a good polish and hopefully try and make a habit of it.

We don't need tins of wax and felt cloths, just some simple milk and honey. This polish is also a good quick fix if you suddenly need to dash somewhere special and you think your skin could do with a quick lift.

A teaspoon of honey and a teaspoon of full cream milk is all you need. Mix together in a little bowl. Use a cotton ball to rub the mixture generously all over your face and neck. Leave on for at least 15 minutes. Rinse off and moisturise as normal.

This should give your face a real good shine for the weekend and an ageless number plate!

ANTI-AGEING AVOCADO

Time flies ever so quickly. Like it or not, we are getting older every day. However, I have always believed that you are only as old as you feel. Feeling young on the inside is a state of mind each individual has to work on. While you work on that, you can also very quickly whip up an anti-ageing facemask to take care of your skin on the outside!

After a good cleanse, a replenishing facemask will help to nourish and rejuvenate the skin.

Avocado is a very nourishing vegetable packed full with antioxidants. Its oils are very anti-ageing and a good way to keep those wrinkles at bay. It is a real treat for dry or mature skin.

For this mask, you will simply need half an Avocado and a teaspoon of Honey.

Take out the contents of half an avocado; mash it up with a fork in a little bowl or a hand-held blender. Add a teaspoon of Honey. Mix the paste until it is nice and smooth.

Gently rub the mixture in circular motion all over your face. Leave on for about 15 to 20 minutes. The longer you leave it on, the better the results

Wipe off with a damp face cloth or wash off with warm water.

Your skin will feel soft to the touch after this.

Always remember that if it is not good enough to eat, it is certainly not good enough to go on your skin.

BEAT LARGE PORES WITH EGGS

I have always said that the refrigerator and your kitchen cupboard hold the key to amazing skin! Always rummage through your fridge and cupboard for yoghurts, old bottles of honey, oats, fruits and veg that you can whip up a facemask or scrub with.

I've had a few questions on how to treat skin with large pores. A good egg mask will do the trick as this will tighten as well as draw impurities out of the skin.

Simply beat a cold egg with a teaspoon of clean water added to it. Gently spread the mix all over your face. Allow to dry. When dry, the skin becomes very taut.

Leave on for 10-15 minutes, then rinse off with warm water, and pat dry. The pores become visibly smaller and the skin will feel taut and clean. Leave skin to breath for a few minutes and then moisturise as normal.

Have fun trying this out!

BRIGHT EYES, CLEAR SKIN, (DESPITE THE ODDS) WITH THE POWER OF LEMONS!

There are times when you feel you have done all you possibly can within your power, to eat well, keep healthy and use the right products; but yet your skin still does not reflect all your hard work!

At times like this, it is worth looking inwards to consider what the problem could really be. There is so much going on in the world around us today that we do not need to look too far for what could be causing some form of stress or the other in our lives. This would be reflected in our eyes and on our skin - the two parts of our body that are not good at camouflaging what we may be going through.

I am no Psychologist, but from experience the first step to keeping those eyes bright and skin glowing even when everything seems to be falling apart, is to look with gratitude at all that IS ACTUALLY GOOD in your life and recognise that there is a lot to be thankful for.

With this positive attitude, start your day with a good cleanse on the inside and the outside;

1. Squeeze half a lemon into a mug of warm water. Brush your teeth first as the acid in the lemon, which could be abrasive. Have this as your first drink for the day. In addition to cleaning your insides and getting you ready for the day, the Lemon is high in Vitamin C, which is very good for the eyes. Vitamin C is found in high concentrations in the tissues of the eye.

   Therefore, a deficiency could result in numerous eye problems such as bleeding in the lids and conjunctiva.

2. After your drink, give your face a good cleanse and a scrub. Put on a brave face (after moisturising of course!), then go out, and face the world believing you have the power to do anything you set your mind to do. Then watch the world fall in line with what you believe.

Remember, half a lemon a day!

CALMING LAVENDER TO SOOTHE THE ITCH

We have had our fair share of bouts of Chicken Pox over the years in our household. Therefore, for our readers who have to deal with this ailment, I thought I should share a helpful remedy for dealing with this whole itchy affair!

This remedy also works for dry, itchy, eczema prone skin.

Firstly, give the child a relaxing bath with a few drops of Lavender Oil added to the water. You simply cannot go wrong with Lavender Oil; it helps relax the nerves and muscles. Most importantly, it cools the skin and relieves the itch. The special properties contained in Lavender Oil also help to heal the skin and prevent the sore spots from getting infected.

To further hasten the healing and relieve the itch, after the bath, put a few drops of the oil on some cotton wool and gently dab this directly onto the spots.

Now, even if you do not ever have the worry of treating Chicken Pox, nothing stops you from still enjoying an indulging soak with some Lavender Oil lavishly sprinkled in the bath water. This will help you relax and soothe your aching muscles after a long week!

CHECK YOUR FIZZ LEVELS

A recent study by US scientists has linked intake of fizzy drinks with violent assaults as reported by The Times and Natural Products Magazine. A cause for great concern I would say…

The research shows that drinking more than 5 cans of fizzy drinks a week is linked to significantly higher levels of violence amongst teenagers. One would imagine that similar effects would in some degree apply to adults too.

This weekend, try out this simple but healthy fizz free drink packed full with antioxidants and vitamins! All you need are:

- Half a glass of cranberry juice
- Half a glass of carrot juice
- A dash of freshly squeezed lemon

Mix these together and you'll have a glass full of a fizz free, power packed health-giving drink.

Cranberry juice is rich in Vitamin C and dietary fibre. Its various health benefits include preventing bladder and urinary tract infections, lowering bad cholesterol, fighting colds and preventing stomach ulcers and cancer. It also helps emulsify fat deposits in the body.

Carrot juice is rich in Vitamins A and C. It helps prevent heart disease, certain cancers, helps with eyesight, diabetes and helps reduce the risk of strokes.

Now which would you rather have; the good health or the violent streak?

CHOCOLATE TREAT FOR YOUR SKIN!

This week, I tried out a new chocolate product – toffee flavoured popcorn covered in chocolate. Really yummy! I feel the need to confess to my trusting readers that I over indulged in this product during the week. It tasted too good to be good for me! In saying that though, it's not always true that anything that's good for you never really tastes good. There are some really amazing tasting foods that are just as good for you on the insides.

The same goes for food for your skin. There are some delicious tasting foods that do wonders for your skin. For instance, milk, honey, chocolate (yes, chocolate!) sugar, yoghurt, eggs and fruits & veggies like lemons, avocados and tomatoes to name a few.

This weekend, let's make a really simple skin brightening face mask packed full with antioxidants and skin rejuvenating properties. You'll only need two simple ingredients, Honey and Cocoa powder. A yummy tasting indulging face mask.

Cocoa is filled with natural antioxidants that help in cell repair and cell damage prevention. Antioxidants help to neutralize free radicals and prevent them from damaging the skin cells.

Honey is a natural antibacterial and antiseptic. Its antioxidants help to eliminate free radicals in the body, they are also part of the nutrient supply for growth of new tissue. It also protects the skin from the sun and helps the skin stay young.

Simply add a teaspoon full of Cocoa powder to 2 teaspoons of Honey. Mix carefully into a paste. Apply onto clean wet skin.

Leave on for 15-20minutes and then gently wash off with warm water.

This mask never fails when you need a quick fix for your skin with intense conditioning.

Have fun with this and have a yummy weekend

CLEANS; NO ADDED PROMISES!

A while ago, I thought with the recession still hitting hard, it was about time, in line with the government, to make some major cuts in the household budget. So, when I went shopping, instead of purchasing one of the leading brands of Laundry Detergent, I opted for the least expensive, no frills alternative.

The message was clear on the pack; Biological Powder. Cleans, no added promises. I thought this was hilarious! It may have been, but the fact I couldn't lose sight of here was that I was actually being told the truth – the message here was:

'This detergent cleans and that's about all it can do for you. It's not promising that your clothes will smell as fresh as summer flowers or that they will come out of the wash as soft as cotton wool; but it certainly cleans.'

So, the question is, do your skincare products tell you the truth? Do they make you presume or blatantly promise healthy skin, with natural toxin free ingredients, with no long term harmful effects in your bloodstream?

Studies have shown that babies are born with 200 chemicals already in their bloodstream. We can't live in ignorance anymore – we really should know what's in our skincare and household products.

This is why I still maintain that if it's not good enough to eat, it's not good enough to go on your skin. Your food and skincare products all end up in the same place; your blood stream!

This week, take some time out and go through the ingredients in the products in your bathroom and do some simple research on the internet on each ingredient.

Have a safe week!

COOK YOUR FOOD, DON'T NUKE IT!

For those of you that have attended my training events, I may be beginning to sound like a broken record on this issue, but this goes to show how dear you all are to me. It's not just what you eat that's important, but also the method of preparation goes a long way to determine the quality of food going into your body. For instance, we all know that steamed for is healthier than fried food.

Let talk about the microwave oven – again! We already know the benefits of the convenience of a microwave oven so this weekend let's do a bit of research on what harmful effects a microwave oven may have long-term.

The picture on the left is my idea of a completely nuked broccoli. It doesn't look appealing on the outside so I don't imagine it will be much different when it gets eaten, or better still offer much nourishment when it gets inside of us.

A study published in the November 2003 issue of The Journal of the Science of Food and Agriculture found that broccoli zapped in the microwave with a little water lost up to 97 percent of the beneficial antioxidant chemicals it contained. By comparison, steamed broccoli lost 11 percent or fewer of its antioxidants.

Dr. Hans Hertel, a Swiss food scientist, carried out some studies on the dangers of the microwave and he concluded that microwave cooking significantly altered foods nutrients resulting in a deterioration of the blood of the participants of the study. His findings showed that microwave cooking resulted in:

- Increased cholesterol levels
- More leukocytes, or white blood cells, which can suggest poisoning
- Decreased numbers of red blood cells

- Production of radiolytic compounds (compounds unknown in nature)
- Decreased haemoglobin levels, which could indicate anaemic tendencies

I think it would be worth doing some more research before warming some milk for your hot cuppa this weekend. While you're doing that, bring out the good old milk pot (which has been a faithful friend for generations now), pour some milk in it, turn on the stove and before you can say 'voila!' you've got some safely warmed up milk!

CRANBERRY TREAT FOR YOUR SKIN

During the Christmas season, your skincare 'treasure chests' (your fridges and kitchen cupboards), will be filled with a few more goodies which you could use for a few new treats for your skin!

Cranberries may one of the goodies in your fridge. Here's how to make a refreshing, anti-ageing, skin tightening Cranberry & Ganoderma Green Tea Face Mask.

Used topically, Cranberries are rich in Vitamin C which helps to build the skins natural collagen keeping the skin healthy and wrinkle free. They are also rich in Vitamin B3 which is very effective in treating acne and Vitamin B5 which helps increase the skins moisture content.

Taken internally, Cranberries are rich in Vitamin C and dietary fibre. They also help prevent bladder and urinary tract infections, lower bad cholesterol, fight colds and help prevent stomach ulcers and cancer. They also help emulsify fat deposits in the body - handy after Christmas meals!

And for your Ganoderma Green Tea, Ganoderma is an ancient Chinese red mushroom that for thousands of years was given to the Emperors for longevity. It was popularly known as "The Elixir of Youth" or "The Immortality Herb"! Green Tea is popularly known for its anti-ageing properties. It contains Polyphenols which go through your blood stream to your skin and help slow down the signs of ageing

For this special Christmas recipe, you'll simply need:

1 cup of Fresh Cranberries

2 Ganoderma Green Tea Bags

2 cups of water

Boil the cranberries in the water for 20 minutes and then add the Ganoderma Green Tea Bags. After this has cooled down a bit, take the tea bags out and use a fork to crush the cranberries to a pulp. Gently rub the cooled pulp on clean skin and leave on for 15 to 20 minutes. Wipe off with a damp face cloth.

Leftovers can be kept in the fridge and used again.

DEFY AGE WITH GREEN TEA & GANODERMA

I've always believed Nature has given us everything we need to keep us healthy and happy on Planet Earth. I guess Mother Nature must've known we would also want to defy time and look younger with every passing day. Well, guess what? She has provided Ganoderma Lucidum (The King of Herbs) and Green Tea to help us defy time!

Green Tea is popularly known for its anti-ageing properties. When you drink it, the Polyphenols in the tea leaves go through your blood stream to your skin and help slow down the signs of ageing.

Ganoderma is an ancient Chinese red mushroom that for thousands of years was given to the Emperors for longevity. It was popularly known as "The Elixir of Youth" or "The Immortality Herb"!

In a United States Patented invention (US Patent No. 7060286 B2 June 13 2006) it was shown that Ganoderma helps protects against the degeneration of skin cells. The related studies showed that Ganoderma helped to smoothen the skin, reduce wrinkles and had age defying properties.

Now that sounds like Botox to me, but without injections and the difficulty of raising your eyebrows!

Optimum benefits can be achieved both by drinking and topical application of the herb.

So, let's make a 'Natural Botox' Face Mask.

You will need 4 teabags of Ganoderma Infused Green Tea.

4 teaspoons of Manuka Honey.

Open up 4 teabags of Ganoderma & Green Tea and grind in a dry food blender into a fine powder.

Add 4 teaspoons of Honey. Mix together till you have a dark paste. Apply to clean face and leave on for 20 minutes. Wash off with warm water and voila! The beginning of a new you!!

DIY SPA FOOT SCRUB!

We have to be a bit more innovative on how we tell our loved ones they are special without necessarily spending too much money.

Sometimes, spending money can be a way of passing the buck to someone else to do a job we could easily have done ourselves. Then again, we don't have to wait for birthdays, anniversaries or special occasions to get our message out to loved ones; or it could even be a special treat for you after a long week. We do need to show ourselves some love too!

So, this weekend, let's roll up our sleeves and give ourselves or someone special the gift of a sweet smelling natural foot scrub!

For this we will need:

- 2 tablespoons of Soft Brown sugar
- 1 table spoon of Extra Virgin Olive Oil
- 1 tablespoon of Honey
- 5 drops of Lavender oil. Mix together in a little bowl.

Soak feet in a large bowl of warm water with a few drops of Lavender oil added to the water. After soaking for about 10 to 15 minutes, rub the mixture all over the feet and ankles with circular movements for a few minutes. Rinse in the water, pat dry and moisturise.

Now put your feet up and have a lovely weekend

EAT YOUR WAY TO YOUTHFULNESS!

Real beauty starts from the inside. This means whatever you put into your body is a determining factor as to how your appearance turns out. Your skin reflects almost everything going on in your life.

 If you are happy and healthy or stressed and overworked, your skin mirrors this to the world. The skin is usually soft and smooth when it is well cared for, or dry and flaky when being taken for granted. Thankfully, the skin renews itself every seven to ten weeks, so it's never too late to start taking good care of your skin.

Having said that, the younger you are when you start taking good care of your skin, the better your skin will turn out to be later in life.

Drinking a lot of water, fresh fruits and vegetables will leave you looking young and healthy. Water helps to cleanse the body of toxins and keeps the skin glowing and well hydrated. Water in itself is a health and beauty tonic. At least eight glasses of water a day would be just right.

A raw food diet will keep you trim, healthy and make your cells grow younger.

The extreme temperatures of cooked food tend to damage your insides just as much as the weather damages the unprotected parts of your body. The stomach enzymes are also adversely affected by hot food and drink. As a result of this, you become deficient in nutrients as your body is unable to extract these nutrients from your digestive tract.

Cooking destroys the enzymes, minerals and vitamins in your food. Furthermore, any process which turns your food brown produces carcinogenic compounds. Try and have at least half of your food raw and you will experience amazing changes.

This week eat raw; you'll actually enjoy it!

Exercise your way to younger skin

I've been doing a lot of walking this week. Not by choice, but it's been fantastic! I feel a lot lighter (don't ask why!) and more energetic. There's no doubt that exercise does wonders for our body. That has been proven time and time again, so I don't need to mention any studies that have been carried out in this regard.

The exciting thing also is that when you exercise, the body's circulation is increased. This goes a long way to improve the appearance of the skin, giving the skin a nice glow.

It also encourages detoxification in the body flushing out toxins especially when you sweat.

Through all this, there is also a process of cell renewal going on. I don't know about yours, but cell renewal means rejuvenation in my books!

This week, don't stay indoors, have a nice walk about, walk to shops instead of driving, have a run in the park and have a vibrant week!

FOODS THAT HEAL: CARROTS

What's in a carrot? Its sweet, it's crunchy and it's loved by rabbits, but sometime the immense benefits of carrots are understated. The Carrot can be used in different ways to get the most of its health benefits. It can be eaten, drank as a juice or its oil used topically on the skin.

Apart from carrots high amounts of Beta-Carotene, carrots also contain a compound called Falcarinol which protect carrots from fungal diseases.

Scientists have investigated this compound extensively. Published studies have suggested that Falcarinol could prevent the development of cancer. Up until recently, it was not known what element of this exceptional vegetable these special cancers had fighting properties.

Carrots also help to cleanse the skin as they are a good detoxifier for the liver – a cleansed liver means less acne! They also have anti-ageing properties as the Beta-Carotene helps to fight cell damage.

Other benefits can be derived from Carrot Oil which is a skin rejuvenator. The oil encourages skin reproduction. It also has anti-inflammatory effects, handy for aches and pains. Carrot Oil also protects the skin from the damaging effects of the sun - Natures very own sun cream!

So, to stay rejuvenated from the inside out, nibble away on some carrots, drink some carrot juice and lavish its oil on your skin – Again, just one of the gifts from Nature's bounty!

FOODS THAT HEAL: GREEN TEA

If we go by the notion (which I strongly believe) that whatever you put on your skin eventually ends up in your bloodstream, then one food I certainly wouldn't mind going into my blood stream is Green Tea!

Green Tea is popularly known for its anti-ageing properties. When you drink it, the Polyphenols in the tea leaves go through your blood stream to your skin and help slow down the signs of ageing.

Green Tea is also packed full with anti-oxidants! Studies have shown that the antioxidants found in Green Tea are over 100 times more effective in neutralizing free radicals than vitamin C, and 25 times more powerful than vitamin E.

The most important antioxidant contained in it is EGCG (epigallocatechin gallate) which is said to reduce cellular damage that could lead to cancer.

It goes without saying that optimum benefits can be achieved both by drinking and topical application of the herb.

So, this weekend let's make a 'Green Tea Skin Toner'. This not only tones the skin and leaves it refreshed and vitalized after cleansing, but if you put some in a nice little spray bottle, you could gently spray those wrinkles away!

Put a teabag of Green Tea in a jug and pour in the equivalent amount of a cup of boiling water. Leave to sit until water cools down completely. Pour into a spray bottle and store in the fridge. After washing your face, spray all over face and neck and let it dry on your skin. Moisturise your skin as normal.

GIVE YOUR HAIR A TREAT

Like the rest of our body, our hair needs daily TLC. However, we tend to ignore the health of our hair so long as it can get us through to the next trip to the barbers or hairdressers. We forget that if our skin needs nourishment daily, so does our scalp – it's still all part of our skin.

You may notice that the skin on your forehead gets slightly dry if your scalp is dry. This is simply because it's all one continuous covering of skin and every inch of it needs special care.

As obvious as it may sound to some of you (not everyone does it) Hair and Scalp Oiling is an excellent treatment for dry hair. It helps promote natural hair growth, relieves itchy scalp and helps with hair loss and the retention of the hairs natural moisture. It also adds shine and lustre to the hair. The process of massaging the scalp is relaxing and encourages blood circulation which in effect stimulates hair growth.

This weekend, try out this simple recipe for Hair Growth:

- Thyme essential oil - 2 drops
- Cedarwood essential oil - 2 drops
- Lavender essential oil -3 drops
- Rosemary essential oil -3 drops (this oil should be omitted for people with low blood pressure)
- Jojoba oil - ½ teaspoon
- Grapeseed oil - 4 teaspoons

Mix the first four oils (the essential oils) together in a little glass jar. Then add the Jojoba and Grapeseed oils and mix together.

Oil the scalp using a small amount at a time so the hair doesn't get too greasy. Massage into the scalp for 2-5minutes. Repeat as often as possible preferably every night.

Get mixing and massaging!

HEAVEN SCENT, NATURE'S SCENT

Have you ever worried about what may be in your perfumes or colognes or have you had an allergic reaction in some way or the other to the chemicals and alcohol contained in them?

This morning, I dabbed on a few drops of Neroli Oil behind my ears and it smelt really good - so I thought I should share this.

You too can enjoy the sweet smell of a home- made fragrance without the worries of its chemical content.

Essential oils are Natures gifts of perfumes to us. It's just about putting them together to suit your 'smell buds'!

A simple musky perfume for men would need:

10 drops of Lavender Oil

20 drops Coriander Oil

22 drops Sandalwood Oil

5 drops Frankincense Oil

100ml Jojoba Oil

And for the ladies, a simple sensual perfume would need:

5 drops of Coriander Oil

6 drops Bergamot Oil

4 drops Neroli Oil

1 drop Jasmine Blend

10ml Jojoba Oil

Mix all the oils together and pour into a little dark bottle. Shake well before use. Rub in a little drop on your pressure points and enjoy the sweet smell of your home-made fragrance.

HERBAL SPA TREAT AT HOME

After a long week, it's only natural that you'll need to unwind one way or another. There's nothing quite like the pleasure of a long warm unwinding soak after a really tiring week. One weekend, give yourself an Herbal Spa Treat at home to soothe those tired muscles.

Most of the ingredients for this treat can be obtained from your local Natural Health Shop or check the resources page at the end of the book for more information on where to get your Herbs from.

Chamomile helps to soothe the muscles and softens the skin. Comfrey and Marigold both have great healing properties.

Lavender is very relaxing and also helps to soothe headaches.

Always check for contraindications and do a patch test to check for skin sensitivity before using any essential oils.

RECIPE:

Put 50g of an equal mixture of the following into a jug:

Dried Chamomile

Comfrey

Marigold

Pour in a pint (600ml) of boiling water and leave to infuse for 30mins.

Run your bath. Strain the infusion through a sieve and pour into the bath water. Add 5-10 drops of Lavender Oil in the bath water.

For this soak, do not add soap to your bath as this will coat your skin and therefore preventing the herbs from penetrating the pores of your skin. Now get a nice book and step into your well-deserved treat.

For health and safety reasons, please don't fall asleep!

HONEY FOR YOUR LIPS IN COLD, DRY WEATHER

The weather is slowly getting cold and dry where I am. That time of the year is slowly and surely creeping up on us. Our skin takes the brunt of harsh weather conditions whether hot, dry, wet or cold and that includes our lips. It's important that we take care of our lips as we do to the rest of our skin to protect it against the elements.

Here's a recipe for a Honey & Rose Lip Balm and then some handy tips for the season ahead: (You can get all the ingredients from your local Health Store)

1 tbsp Rosehip Seed Oil

I tbsp Calendula Oil

5 tbsp Sweet Almond Oil

1 drop Honey

1 tbsp of Beeswax pellets

2 Vitamin E capsules

5 drops of Rose Oil

Use a double boiler or put a small saucepan into another with hot water in the bigger saucepan.

Pour in the oils, add the honey, beeswax and stir gently. While the beeswax is melting, prick open the Vitamin E capsules and squeeze into the mix. When beeswax has fully melted, take off from the heat, put the 5 drops of rose oil and stir until it all mixed in. Pour into little glass jars and leave to cool and set.

Handy tips:

- Keep your skin hydrated and drink at least 2litres of water everyday
- Use nutrient rich oils on the skin straight after a shower such as Olive, Avocado and Sweet Almond Oils.
- Use a good hydrating face mask/scrub at least once a week to get rid of dead, flaky skin – you can contact me to make you some!
- Moisturise day and night with a natural, rich moisturiser.

So, don't leave it too late, start getting ready for the cold dry weather now.

HOW CLEAN IS YOUR MAKE-UP?

Make-up is a lot like your clothes. It goes on after your outsides have been cleansed. Surely you wouldn't apply your make-up just before you cleanse your face or just before a shower!

After making an effort to ensure your outsides are squeaky clean (and assuming that your insides are also clean), it's important that the make-up you put on your skin is also clean.

I've always maintained that there is no excuse for not taking the time to read the ingredients of any product that goes on your skin as it eventually ends up in your blood stream. The way you read the nutritional contents of your food items when you go grocery shopping should also be done for your make-up and skin products. Educate yourself on the harmful ingredients contained in these products. It's been said that every year our bodies absorb 2 kilograms of chemicals from chemicals found in skincare, make-up and hair products.

There are certain ingredients you should always be on the lookout for. Clean make-up should be free from synthetic chemicals and harmful ingredients. Nitrosating agents such as paraben preservatives are but a few of such ingredients to be cautious of.

If you would like some more information on ingredients to watch out for in your make-up and other skincare products, send me a message on our Facebook page https://www.facebook.com/RichesInEden requesting a Toxic Ingredients Directory to be sent out to you…. Then make the decision yourself!

IT MAY BE WINTER OUTSIDE....

The year was 1973, and they were called 'Love Unlimited', for those who were trying really hard to remember the group that sang this! It's snowing where I am and it's all white and beautiful everywhere; But with the beauty of the snow, come the colds, sniffles and chesty coughs.

If it's cold and wintery outside wherever you are, this weekend, bring the warmth of spring in by making yourself a mug of freshly squeezed lemon juice in some warm water, with a dash of honey.

And to keep your chest and congested sinuses clear, have a Eucalyptus Face Steam.

Get a large bowl of hot water and put in a few drops of Eucalyptus Oil in the water.

Carefully put your face over the bowl covering your head with a towel. Inhale the steam for at least 3-5minutes at a time. Repeat until the water cools down.

Gently pat your face dry.

Asides from clearing your chest, this treatment also helps to open up the pores and detoxifies the skin on your face. So, make the most of it by giving your face a good scrub with our 4-in-1 edible and nourishing Facial Scrub. Now curl up and enjoy your warm mug of Lemon juice and Honey (if it hasn't gone cold already!)

So, 'it may be zero degrees with the snow falling down', but you can still have a warm restful weekend!

JUST GIVE LOVE!

'Just Give Love' – the words of wise counsel given to me this morning. If we could simply give a bit more love, we would find solutions to many of the situations we find ourselves in daily.

This brings to mind famous sayings such as 'love your neighbour as yourself' or 'do unto others as you would have them do unto you'. With these two sayings, it is assumed that we love ourselves – we have to love ourselves to be able to show this same love to our 'neighbours' or to others.

You may wonder what this has to do with health and beauty. It has a lot do with it. How do you show love to yourself? Do you take care of your body so it stays healthy for a long time to come? Do you eat right? Do you take care of your skin which gives you protection from the outside world? Do you clean and nourish it? How often?

How often do you spend time with yourself and give yourself some 'me time'? Spending some quiet time alone goes a long way to help keep you calm, focused and reinvigorated ready to face the race out there.

This weekend, ask yourself these questions, think about giving yourself some love and then pass this love on to others.

So, give some love and have a lovely weekend!

LET'S GET LIPPY

Considering the fact that our lips have the thinnest skin on our bodies and have the least natural moisture, they don't always get the right care and attention they deserve.

Care doesn't mean the rigorous rubbing of lip balm during dry weather or a quick dash of lipstick for the ladies as you rush out the door in the morning. Like it or not, care of the lips should be part of your skincare regime.

So here are some handy tips for your 'lip care' regime:

- Moisturise your lips daily with a good lip balm that is free of Menthol and Camphor as these tend to dry out the lips
- To get rid of dry, dead skin on the lips, rub in some Petroleum Jelly or lip balm and then gently brush the lips with a soft tooth brush or a damp flannel
- The lips are prone to sunburn so use a lip balm that contains sunscreen
- For quick hydration for overly dry lips, gently rub in the contents of a pierced Vitamin E capsule on the lips
- For the ladies, avoid using lip sealants as they contain a lot of chemicals. They also dry the lips and are not suitable for sensitive skin
- To treat stained lips, regularly rub the lips with Olive Oil. This also helps to keep them moisturized
- If you've got cracks at the corners of your lips, you may be Vitamin B deficient. Try eating so more whole grain food, red meat and green veggies
- A finally those tiny lines around the edge of the lips that show up when a lady's lipstick 'bleeds'! The main culprit for this is smoking.

If you do smoke, try to cut down or quit by the New Year. Line your lips and use a less glossy lipstick that won't 'bleed'. Keep your lips hydrated as stated above.

LOOK YOUNG WITH THE POWER OF GINGER!

I love Ginger in my food. It has a way of turning an otherwise bland and boring dish into an exciting meal! But besides spicing up a dish, Ginger is a superfood with very potent medicinal and skincare properties.

Ginger has traditionally been used to help inflammatory joint diseases such as arthritis. It is also known to help with circulation and therefore promoting cardiovascular health.

Studies have also suggested that Ginger may be useful in keeping cholesterol levels under control, although how this works is not fully understood. Ginger also has warming expectorant action on the upper respiratory tract, good for treating colds and influenza

And for your skin, Ginger helps fight inflammations that could give rise to acne or psoriasis. It's an amazing antioxidant for fighting skin damage thereby slowing down the skins ageing process.

Another fantastic thing about Ginger is that it smoothens and tones the skin and is a very good weapon for fighting age spots – yes, those little brown spots that slowly creep up on you as the years go by!

You can target those age spot by simply rubbing a fresh slice of Ginger directly onto the dark spots 2-3 times a day.

However, the best way to get the full benefit of Ginger internally and externally is to drink it! Cut up a few fresh Ginger slices, put in a mug, pour in some boiling water and let it soak for about

5 to 10 minutes. When it's cooled down a bit, add a little honey and stir well and enjoy.

I have always believed that beauty starts from the inside. What you put into your body (food and cosmetics alike) will have a resultant effect on how your body looks and feels. Every organ in your body is dependent on what goes into the body as a whole; so, you really are 'what you eat' as they say.

CAUTION! Even though Ginger is known to help with nausea, it should still be used with great caution in pregnancy as it's known to stimulate blood flow. Always seek advice from your Medical Practitioner before using any herbs.

NATURAL AFTERSHAVE

Something especially for the men today. Have you ever wondered what it would be like to make your own home-made aftershave? Ok, maybe not. – But here's a simple recipe you could try your hands at this weekend. One of the ingredients is Vodka and I'm hoping that the reason for buying this little bottle of Vodka should be solely for the purpose of making this Aftershave. Promise?

The ingredients you'll need are:

1 ½ Tablespoon of Pure Vodka

8 drops of Sandalwood Essential Oil

3 drops of Neroli Essential Oil

6 ½ Tablespoons of Rose Water

4 Tablespoons of Witch Hazel

Vodka has special healing properties in it. It's a good disinfectant. It's helps combat pimples associated with shaving and it's also a good treatment for infected boils.

Sandalwood has been in use for over 6,000 years. Its oil is warm, soothing and relaxing. A few of its health benefits are that it's anti-septic, anti-inflammatory and is a very good astringent and emollient. Neroli Oil has similar properties too.

Witch Hazel's astringent, anti-viral, anti-septic and anti-inflammatory properties make it a good treatment for cuts & bruises and itchy and irritated skin.

Rose Water has soothing, deep cleansing, and skin toning properties. It also tightens the pores and reduces wrinkles. Ensure you use pure Rose Water which can be found in most pharmacies.

To make the Aftershave, get a glass bottle of about 200ml in size and pour in the Vodka. Add the Essential oils and shake well.

Next add the Witch Hazel. Shake well and then add the Rose Water and shake again. Always remember to shake well before use.

And there you have it. Your own home-made Aftershave. These amazing ingredients should get your skin looking a million dollars this weekend!

Have a lovely one.

NATURAL SKIN LIGHTENER…. ONLY IF YOU MUST!

The grass is always greener on the other side, they say. If you've got light skin, you may want it a shade darker and vice versa. Most times it's safer to just let things be. However, there may be situations where we have dark patches of skin that we're not comfortable with. If this is the case, I believe if you must lighten your skin, do it the safe way…. chemical free.

This is a quick recipe for a Skin Lightening Face Mask, which with regular use (say once or twice a week), may help lighten skin with dark patches.

Wash your face before using this mask.

You'll need One Lime, One Tomato and about a teaspoon or less of flour to thicken your mask.

Chop up a medium sized tomato and pop into the blender. Squeeze the juice of one lime and add to the blender. Mix this together. Pour out into a little bowl and thicken with a bit of flour. Rub this in circular motion all over the face or area to be lightened. Leave on for about 20minutes and then rinse off with cold water. Moisturise your skin as normal.

If you've got really sensitive skin, don't leave on for too long as the lime may sting a bit.

Don't expect overnight results. A bit of patience would come in handy!

Another good thing about this mix is that you can enjoy a nice smoothie if you have any leftovers in the blender - without the flour of course!

NATURALLY HEALTHY AGELESS SKIN

Whatever your age, a good skin care regime will help heal whatever damage or trauma your skin may have gone through. We can all have wonderful skin if we make the right choices in our lifestyle.

Using skincare products made from natural ingredients, having a diet rich in the essential fatty acids such as in flax seed oil and olive oil will all help to maintain healthy skin. Adequate sleep and exercise also play a great role in achieving beautiful healthy skin.

The trick to a younger look is to have healthy glowing skin. To achieve this, follow a simple skin care regime.

Your simple skin care steps are:

- Gentle cleansing – Always cleanse your face and neck in the morning and at night. This helps to get rid of accumulated dead cells and all the grime picked up in the air. A natural soap or cleanser is advisable.
- Toning – A good toner helps to tighten and tone the pores of the skin. Always use one that is alcohol-free and infused with essential oils as this will not be harsh on the skin.
- Day time moisturizing – A light or rich skin moisturizer depending on your skin type will keep your skin's moisture locked in all day. Keep your lips moist especially when out in the sun
- Night time moisturizing – At night, a rich moisturiser will rejuvenate and hydrate your skin while you sleep. Use a moisturiser formulated with essential oils
- Exfoliants or Scrubs – Once a week, exfoliate your skin with a good skin scrub. Keep your scrub as simple and as natural as possible. Exfoliants help to remove dead cells from the skins surface and also encourage blood circulation and production of new cells. This helps to give the skin a healthy glow.

Naturally healthy skin should be free from harmful chemicals, well hydrated from within and without and nourished with a balanced diet and wise food choices.

And finally, a positive outlook to life, a pleasant disposition and a smile will contribute greatly to keeping you ageless from the inside out!

THE POWER OF A SIMPLE ONION!

There are a lot of amazing Super- foods out there such as the Ganoderma (Reishi), Goji berries, Noni fruit and Acai berries - and so it's very easy not to notice the not so 'super food' staring you in the face in your kitchen everyday – The simple onion!

Yes, the simple lonely onion that is always there even when you run out of salt!

Did you know that the onion is the richest dietary source of Quercetin? Quercetin is a potent antioxidant that has been directly linked to inhibiting stomach cancer.

Its strong antioxidant properties help protect the body from cancer by reducing damage to our DNA in the cells. An important point to note is that Quercetin is found in most onions e.g. shallots, yellow and red onions but NOT IN WHITE ONIONS. This may be a good time to switch your onion preference!

The Quercetin in the onions also helps with thinning of blood, heart problems, lowering of cholesterol and increasing good cholesterol. It helps fight asthma and bronchitis, diabetes, infections and it acts like an antihistamine for hay fever.

You can bet that I'm not done until I've told you its benefits for your skin!

Many commercial creams use onion extract as an anti-inflammatory in their creams to treat scars. The onion juice is also handy for treating

warts and freckles. Soak a slice of onion in cider vinegar overnight, tape on to the warts and watch them go in weeks!

Onions are very rich in Sulphur, a vital mineral for the health of our skin, hair and nails. Rubbing onion juice into the scalp at least 3 times a week is believed to help with hair growth, restoring hair follicles and promoting strong hair. I'm going to try this one out. If anyone is happy to try this out with me for a month, so we can compare notes, give me a shout!

So, word of advice for the weekend - treat that last onion, lost somewhere between all the potatoes in your kitchen cupboard with a little bit more respect – it's a true life saver!

RAINBOW COLOURS FOR YOUR SKIN!

It may sound child-like, but your skin could really do with a good splash of rainbow colours to brighten it up. By this I mean a colour representing a vital food ingredient for your skin and over-all health!

The phytochemicals responsible for the bright colours in fruits and veg keep us healthy and protect us from cell damage.

I had to go through my little daughter's books to remember the colours in the right order! Here goes:

Red: Red fruits and veg are coloured by the plant pigment 'Lycopene'. Lycopene can be found in high quantities in tomatoes. It also occurs in Watermelon and Pink Grapefruits. Lycopene protects the skin from environmental damage and helps improve the skins texture

Orange/Yellow: Orange and yellow foods are coloured by the pigment 'Carotenoids' which as the name implies can be found in foods such as carrots. It can also be found in Bell Peppers, Sweet Potatoes and Papaya. Amongst its many other benefits which I've spoken about in previous newsletters, Carotenoids help protect the skin from sun damage

Green: Green foods get their colour from the pigment 'Chlorophyll'. Most of us should remember that from science classes in school (if you're having trouble remembering, call me and order some Gingko – very good for the memory!). Chlorophyll can be found in dark leafy vegetables like spinach. It helps detox the system. A well detoxed colon keeps you less prone to Acne!

 Blue/Indigo/Violet: And finally, the blue, purply foods. The blue pigment is 'Anthocyanins' found in foods such as Blueberries, Grapes, Raisins and Eggplant. Anthocyanins are also known as 'The Colour

of Youth'! This antioxidant helps protect the skin from cell damage,
reduces skin inflammation and helps stabilize collagen in the skin – in
simple language - Blueberries not Botox!

SAVE AN ANIMAL: MAKE YOUR SKINCARE PRODUCTS!

If skincare products were edible, then animal testing would not be necessary. True or false? If we could 'eat' these products, then what's there to test? Calorie content? I reckon that Skincare products are tested to find out what negative effect the products could have on animals (to prevent this happening to humans); and not to find out if the poor rabbits wrinkles will disappear after a few weeks of application of the 'Wonder Cream'!

I don't have any pets and I don't lay claims to being involved in any animal rights activities - I'm just simply talking 'Edible Skincare'. Why infuse a Skin Lotion with chemicals when it can be infused with Nature's bounty?

It's about time we took as much control over what we put on our skin as we do what we eat. So, as you shop for healthy ingredients to make your food at home, do the same for your skin. If we don't start taking control now, there will come a time when it will be too late to repair the damage done by the toxins we've slowly put into our bodies. As we strive to keep to our 'five a day' fruits and vegetables, please make the same effort for your skin, otherwise we may very well be fighting a losing battle however much fruit and veg we consume.

The first step towards taking control is by learning how to make simple products for your skin. Nothing expensive or time consuming – just simple products that will do what Nature put them there to do for you.

STEAM AWAY THE SNIFFLES!

It's that time of the year again… the weather is slowly changing and our bodies are trying really hard to adapt to the change.

In come the sniffles, colds, sore throats and congested sinuses. This is just the time for a Steam Treatment to get you up and going!

Get a large bowl of hot water; put 3drops each of Eucalyptus and Peppermint Oils in the water.

Carefully put your face over the bowl covering your head with a towel. Inhale the steam for at least 3-5minutes at a time. Repeat until the water cools down.

Gently pat your face dry.

This treatment helps to clear your sinuses. It also opens up the pores and detoxifies the skin on your face. Make the most of this treatment by cleansing and moisturising your skin afterwards.

And finally, don't forget your citrus fruits for your daily dose of Vitamin C to keep those sniffles at bay!

TAKING THE 'UGH' OUT OF CASTOR OIL!

I don't know about you, but the thought of Castor Oil does not bring back 'pleasant tasting' childhood memories for me. Growing up, my mother gave it to my sister and me whenever she felt we had indulged in too much junk food and needed to clean-out our systems. The intentions were good (oh yes, detox came in many forms back then!) but the taste was worse than 'ugh' with a shiver!!

Now that I'm just a bit older, I've come to really appreciate the potent medicinal and healing properties of Castor Oil.

I have also had to recommend this Oil to a few clients recently and so I felt the need to talk about this oil in a bit more detail, with a simple recipe to try at home.

Castor oil is a pale yellow liquid extracted from castor beans (Ricinus communis). Castor trees are found mainly in the tropics, the Mediterranean and the warmer parts of India. It's medicinal and curative uses date way back to the ancient Egyptian time.

Castor oil has the ability to penetrate the skin deeply working on fine lines and wrinkles better than almost any anti-ageing cream you could buy. It's an excellent source of Vitamin E, antioxidants and triglyceride fatty acids essential for skin health. It also has antiviral and antibacterial properties.

It also has anti-inflammatory properties and is a good treatment for spots, blemishes and acne. It helps the skins production of collagen and Elastin.

I found out recently that castor oil is a good treatment for skin moles and benign skin growth. So, if you've got those annoying dark spots on your skin, give Castor Oil a go for a short while and see.

For the hair, Castor oil helps with scalp infections associated with hair loss. It also strengthens the hair roots and promotes hair growth.

Castor Oil makes a fantastic cleanser for oily skin. Rub into skin and clean off with cotton wool balls. It takes all your make-up off as it cleans.

Better still, make a simple facial scrub and give your skin a new glow this weekend. You'll need:

2 level tablespoons of soft brown sugar

1 tablespoon of Pure Cold Pressed Castor Oil

1 teaspoon of Extra Virgin Olive Oil

1 tablespoon of Honey

Mix all the ingredients together into a nice paste. Rub all over wet face scrubbing as you go along. Leave on for about 20minutes and then rinse off with warm water. Dab skin dry and don't rub your skin.

THE POWER OF HEMP SEED OIL

For years, Hemp Seed Oil has been treated as some sort of villain considering its source. I consistently maintain that every herb, seed or plant is an answer to a problem, even if it's a problem yet unknown. In my studies and research in herbal and natural remedies, I have found that the 'not knowing' what is out there available for us is a bigger problem than all the issues life throws at us.

I'm not giving any recipes but rather I want to draw your attention to the power of Hemp Seed Oil.

Studies have shown that Hemp Seed Oil contains all the essential amino acids and fatty acids necessary for human life. It also has a rare protein- Globule Edestin, which is similar to the globulin found in the human blood plasma. This protein was discovered in Hemp Seed as far back as 1881.

Hemp Seed Oil has is the richest single source of essential oil. Its amazing properties could help repair damaged immune systems.

A few other benefits of this oil when taken internally include, smoother skin, increased vitality, enhanced immune function, helps fight infections and allergies, helps in the formation of cell membrane, keeps the arteries supple amongst so much more!

Thankfully, we've got the internet, so you don't have to rely solely on my words. This weekend, take some time out to research the wealth of health benefits in this oil. You will also find out why goodness of this oil this has been kept very quiet over the years.

A verse in the Bible says, 'my people perish for lack of knowledge'. Let's stop all the 'perishing' in its tracks and open our minds to what nature has made available for us out there. Let's put all the knowledge to good use so we can live longer healthier lives.

THE SECRET TO SHINY HAIR

I recently got my hair 'locked' and I'm already missing the fact that I can't condition my hair just yet so I don't get the 'locks' untangled. This is however a really irresistible recipe for shiny hair that I'm giving a lot of thought without the knowledge of my hair dresser! Try this especially if your hair has had a bad stint with chemical treatments and hair dyes.

The ingredients are:

1 Avocado

1 Banana

2 teaspoons of Extra Virgin Olive Oil

1 Egg

The Avocado is my favourite ingredient for an anti-wrinkle mask and its nutrients and natural fats have amazing benefits for the hair as well. Avocados are rich in Vitamin A, D and E. These vitamins help to rebuild the hair and encourage re-growth in cases of hair loss.

Bananas are rich in Potassium and vitamins such as Vitamin B. The Vitamin B in bananas helps to add moisture to the scalp of the hair. Bananas help to soften the hair and protect dyed and treated hair from further damage. It helps the hair retain its elasticity thereby protecting it from breakage and split ends and also giving the hair strength, shine and volume.

We've talked about the benefits of Olive oil for the skin several times. Olive oil helps to cleanse, nourish and condition the hair and scalp. It also helps improve the elasticity of the hair.

Raw eggs have a high concentration of proteins and vitamins that help to nourish and strengthen the hair follicles. They also help to add shine and volume to the hair leaving it with a nice texture.

Put all the ingredients in a blender and blend till nice and smooth. Rub in all over the hair massaging the hair follicles as you go along. Leave in for about 15 to 20 minutes and shampoo off as normal. When washing off, remember not to use hot water so you don't end up with scrambled eggs in your hair!

THINGS LOOK BETTER IN THE MORNING!

Most things look better in the morning! A mountainous situation doesn't seem so much of a hill after you've slept over it; that daunting piece of work seems less daunting after a good night's rest.

The same goes for your skin. Your skin really should look its best after a good clean and a good night's rest.

At the end of the day before going to bed, mix a teaspoon of honey and a teaspoon of fresh milk together; rub this all over your face and leave on for ten minutes.

Next give your face a good scrub with a warm, damp face flannel. Rinse off the milk and honey mix and dab off any excess water still leaving your face slightly moistened.

Finally, as your night oil, gently rub a few drops of Extra Virgin Olive into your skin. This should nourish your skin as you sleep.

When you wake up the next morning, you'll take one look in the mirror and go: "things sure do look good in the morning"!

TREATING HAIR LOSS

Like the rest of our body, our hair needs daily TLC. However, we tend to ignore the health of our hair so long as it can get us through to the next trip to the barbers or hairdressers. We forget that if our skin needs nourishment daily, so does our scalp – it's still all part of our skin.

You may notice that the skin on your forehead gets slightly dry if your scalp is dry. This is simply because it's all one continuous covering of skin and every inch of it needs special care.

As obvious as it may sound to some of you (not everyone does it) Hair and Scalp Oiling is an excellent treatment for dry hair. It helps promote natural hair growth, relieves itchy scalp and helps with hair loss and the retention of the hairs natural moisture. It also adds shine and lustre to the hair. The process of massaging the scalp is relaxing and encourages blood circulation which in effect stimulates hair growth.

A simple recipe for a Blend for Hair Growth is as follows:

- Thyme essential oil - 2 drops
- Cedarwood essential oil - 2 drops
- Lavender essential oil -3 drops
- Rosemary essential oil -3 drops (this oil can be omitted for people with low blood pressure)
- Jojoba oil - ½ teaspoon
- Grapeseed oil - 4 teaspoons

Mix the first four oils in a little glass jar and mix well. Add the Jojoba and Grapeseed oils and mix together.

Use a little at a time so the hair doesn't get too greasy. Massage into the scalp for 2-5minutes every night.

Also try and relax a bit more. Take life a bit less seriously as stress is a big cause of hair loss.

Learn to take one day at a time…

TURNING BACK TIME FOR YOUR SKIN

Time goes by ever so quickly. With time going by so quickly, so does the elasticity of our skin. This weekend, let's take control of things and help our skin rebuild it collagen levels with a very simple treatment.

Collagen is the most abundant natural protein found in the body. It makes up at least 75% of the body's skin tissue. It could also be described as the skins building blocks and is important for overall health of the skin. The body's collagen levels have been said to slowly diminish from the age of 25 onwards.

The presence of Collagen helps to plump up the skin, reduces lines, wrinkles and generally improves the skin's elasticity. The resultant effect being younger looking radiant skin.

The best way to restore collagen levels in the skin is by naturally helping the skins ability to produce its own collagen. Collagen could be applied topically, but apart from the great expense, sometimes the molecules of the topical Collagen could be too large for the skin to absorb.

This weekend go into your local department store and simply buy a jar of Manuka Honey! Manuka Honey is produced by honey bees that get their nectar from the flowers of the manuka bush. The strength in each jar is measured in UMF Levels and I would always advice any strength from 10+.

Amongst its numerous health properties, Manuka honey has the ability to heal the skin and may also help stimulate the skins process of producing its own collagen.

First, wash your face and then rub about a spoonful of manuka honey all over your slightly wet face. Leave on for about 30minutes.

For even better results, for the last 10 to 15minutes, steam your face over a bowl of warm water or place a warm towel over your face changing the towel as it cools down.

Do this at least once to twice a week. If you've got a bit more time, then 3 times a week would be fantastic!

Take a close up 'before' picture of your skin just before you start this treatment and an 'after' picture in 4weeks time. Let your skin do the talking!

WATER FOR HEALTHY SKIN

Nothing beats water to keep healthy and hydrated. To keep things from getting boring, you can flavour your water with a dash of freshly squeezed lemon juice. The whole idea really is to keep drinking and make a habit of it!

Today, make the most of water. After you've washed your face, give your skin a good steam.

You'll need a bowl of hot water with a few drops of Lavender Oil. Lean over the bowl and cover your head with a towel. Do this for a few minutes and gently dab your face dry.

Steaming the skin helps to open up your pores and also hydrates your skin. It's also detox for your skin.

After you've steamed, your skin is now ready for whatever nourishment you feed it with. Moisturise your skin as normal and then sit down and enjoy a tall glass of water – one of your eight for the day!

FEED YOUR SKIN FROM THE RICHES IN EDEN

Nothing beats knowing what's going on your skin. Sometimes, even with the natural skincare products in the shops, there could still be some ingredients you are allergic to. These ingredients could be safe but just don't agree with you. Just as it's good to be in control of what you eat, it's also good to be in control of what goes on your skin.

Experiment with food on your skin. You will be amazed at how your skin will respond.

For products made from fresh ingredients, make them and use them fresh on the day. You could or keep them in the fridge but only for a few days so you don't have a build up of microbes in it.

For ingredients that are not fresh like oils or dried foods, so long as you don't add water to the composition, chances are that the product will keep for much longer. Water is what triggers the growth of microbes in our products. For instance, how long would a bottle of olive oil, honey or tea last in your kitchen cupboard? At least a year. That's how long your product would last if you keep it dry and away from moisture.

The aim is to use what God has put at our disposal for our body and our skin.

We have to stop poisoning our bodies and that of our families with man-made ingredients with no nutritional value.

Let's stick to Gods original plan for us. His plans for us are always good. Jeremiah 29:11 - For I know the plans I have for you," declares the Lord, "plans to prosper you and not to harm you, plans to give you hope and a future.

If this is His promise for us, why do we walk outside His plans for us and feed our bodies with toxins that could harm us and take away our future?

Handy skincare tips:

- Put some Extra Virgin Olive oil on some cotton wool to take your make-up off. Olive oil is a beauty oil, it nourishes and conditions the skin.
- If your eyes are tired or swollen soak two teabags of green tea in hot water, put it in the fridge to cool and then put over your eyes
- If you run out of deodorant, squeeze some lemon juice and use under your arms. It kills the microbes that cause body odour. Remember that anti-perspirants are not good for you. They block your pores and stop the skin from breathing.
- Grapeseed oil is a light oil, very inexpensive that's very rich in vitamin C. You can use it even if you have oily skin. It evens out your skin tone and tightens the skin.
- Applying Egg white on the skin overnight helps with acne and pimples

Always remember that both your food and your skincare products end up in the same place; your blood stream. So, if your skincare products are not good enough to eat they probably shouldn't go on your skin!

Tap into the resources God has provided for us in Nature and feed your skin and your body the right food

RESOURCES AND REFERENCES

- For any further information on natural health and skincare contact Emma on Facebook at www.facebook.com/RichesInEden
- Environmental Working Group; Body Burden — The Pollution in New-borns. A benchmark investigation of industrial chemicals, pollutants and pesticides in umbilical cord blood. July 14, 2005
- The Bible, NIV Version